Dedicated to

My spiritual master

H.H.Bhakti Raghava Swami

Thankful for the loving support from my family

My yogini wife Sundari Dasi

& my little kids

Bhumikanya and Nemai Gaur Sundar

Healing Mudrās

Heal with the yoga of the hands
with Mudrās for life

Yogi Natarāj

ISBN: 978-1-63625-684-9

Now more than ever, there is a need to focus on self-healing. Mudrās are the best way to self-heal. A combination of mudrās and diet can take us a long way forward to self-healing. Mudrās are so easy to practice, and the results can be realized immediately. From serious health issues to simple day to day illnesses, meditation, visualization of goals, mudrās are useful everywhere.

How to use this book

We have explained the various mudrās in the book in a systematic manner.

1. First, we have introduced the mudrās for the five basic elements. The five elements that govern our body are earth, water, fire, air and ether.

2. Then a combination of these elements which make up the main bodily constituents, Kapha (Earth + Water), Pitta (Fire + Water), and Vāta (Air + Ether) and how they are balanced is explained.

3. Then we have dealt with the five airs and how the airs govern our bodily energy. The five airs are Prāṇa (governs the upward movement of air and energy), Apāna (governs the downward movement of air), Samāna (the fire of digestion), Vyāna (the air which balances everything), Udana (the air in the neck region which governs upward movement).

4

4. Mudrās for Meditation, to purify the nervous system and increase concentration.

5. Mudrās for life — How to achieve our purpose.

6. Mudrās for detoxing the digestive and excretory systems.

7. Mudrās for healing - By learning basic healing mudrās, we can heal any prevalent health issue or bring them under control. The best effect of the mudrās is achieved when we can be quiet and focused on the mudrā taking a deep breath. The beauty of the mudrās is that they are effective whenever they are performed with or without focus, just by the hand positions.

At the end of the book, we have introduced several meditations with a sequence of mudrās for healing and mudrās for life. Once you learn the hand positions properly and practice them in a series, everything becomes sublime.

All the guided mudrā meditations have been converted to guided audio and video mudrās on our website

www.yoginataraj.com/mudra

Table of Contents

Foundational principles of mudrās

Constitution of our body according to Ayurveda

Practice of Mudrās

Mudrās for the life airs

Mudrās for improving heat/digestion

Mudrās for Detox

Mudrās for life

Please read disclaimer in the end before using the book

Why practice mudrās?

In todays world, we are living extremely stressful lives. Whether at work or at home, we face stress in different ways. Stress over a long period of time leads to many psychosomatic diseases which, if not controlled, can lead to chronic lifelong problems. In this seemingly difficult situation, ancient yogic science of the east gives us some good news. Most chronic illnesses can be controlled or healed by the practice of *mudrās* and a proper diet. Our bodies have the capacity to heal themselves. This capacity is re-ignited in the practice of mudrās. It's a beautiful science healing, when understood and practiced, can do wonders. Mudrā means seal. In Sanskrit, the word also relates to mudita, which means "to feel a sense of happiness." Many hundreds of mudrās deal with art, healing, and meditation. This book will deal with only the most essential healing mudrās and various ways we can apply them.

Nādis (or our nervous system)

Our body is a network of gross and subtle nerves. In the Sanskrit language these nerves are called *nādis*. The word nāda means flow, and Nādi is that which facilitates this flow. Our bodies and minds are continually ingesting, digesting, and eliminating waste from the body and minds. It's a flow of traffic. Vāta (A combination of air and ether) carries blood, energy, and oxygen to different parts of the body, and it also eliminates in the form of urine, stool, and sweat. Simultaneously, thoughts and feelings are also carried to the different parts of the body from the mind by a combination of ether and air. Ether carries sound, and the air carries both gross and subtle elements.

Digestion and Excretion

In the body, digestion and excretion are equally important. A disturbance or block in either of these systems causes a problem or disease. Both assimilation and excretion depend on the proper flow of food and air in the nādis or the nerves. When the nerves are blocked or constricted by any means, the current is restricted or blocked, leading to disease. The practice of yoga (which includes the mudrās) keeps the nerves healthy (and open), aiding the proper flow of food, air and thoughts at both the physical and mental levels. This book will specifically deal with the practice of mudrās.

1. *Yogic Mudrās*: Mudrās performed with the entire body
2. *Hasta Mudrās*: Mudrās practiced with the fingers.

In this book, we will cover important *Hasta Mudrās,* healing mudrās with the hands. The yogic mudrās involve physical āsanās and holding them in a proper position. The hand (hasta) mudrās are about the fingers in different hand gestures. These mudrās are very useful when performed with adequate understanding. In this book, we have also added audio and video meditations (links at the end of the book) for different sequences of mudrās for health and meditation. Deep breathing increases the focus on the mudrā and multiplies its effect. The mudrās can be effective otherwise, even if we hold them casually. However, the more we focus on the mudrās with a calm mind combined with deep breathing, the more their effectiveness improves. The mudrās help us at both the physical and mental levels.

Physically they help remove blocks in energy flow by balancing the elements. Mentally, they clear the clutter around the mind, aiding the proper flow of thoughts, giving us mental clarity.

What Mudrās can do and what they cannot

1. Mudrās are very easy to practice.
2. They improve your bodily resistance. With improved resistance power, we can easily overcome any disease.
3. Mudrās have no side effects.
4. Mudrā therapy is safe, and once learned it is literally free of charge.
5. By understanding our bodily consitution (as per Āyurveda), and what we are susceptible, to we use mudrās as a preventive tool.
6. Mudrās can be practiced by anyone, in any condition.
7. Mudrā therapy can be combined advantageously with other forms of treatment: traditional as well as modern. Being a part of yoga and Āyurveda, it goes especially well with Yoga practices and Āyurvedic diet.
8. Mudrās are very effective in dealing with chronic conditions; however, for purely physical debilitating conditions like a fracture, cataract, etc., where surgical or strong physical intervention is required, they work slowly.
9. Mudrās should be preferably practiced on an empty stomach.

Ayurveda
elements

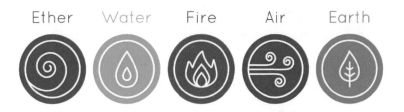

Ether   Water   Fire   Air   Earth

5 Elements of the body

Our body is composed of five elements - Earth, Water, Air, Fire, and Sky/Space and they are represented by the five fingers on our hand. Modern science agrees that different kinds of electromagnetic waves are transmitted from our fingertips. These fingers act like control switches, which can increase (accelerate) or decrease (deccelerate) the influence of a particular element in the body. Each end of a finger is like the end of an electrode; when connected to the proper end, it will complete the circuit, activating a beautiful flow of energy in the body.

Every gesture or mudrā, influences a specific element or a group of elements. It's a science that needs to be understood clearly, and once done, we can logically apply them for therapeutic and meditative purposes. Our body can rejuvenate itself if we position the fingers on both hands for a prescribed period.

The five elements are present in the following order.

1. Thumb - Fire (Agni)
2. Forefinger - Air (Vāyu)
3. Middle Finger - Ether (Ākāsh)
4. Ring Finger - Earth (Prithvi)
5. Little Finger - Water (Jala)

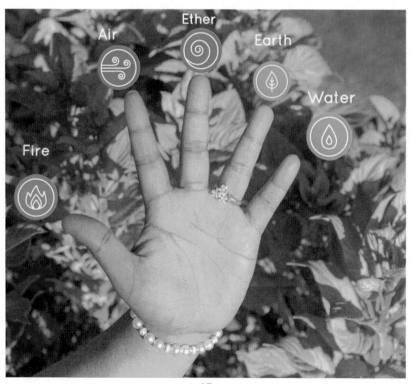

The finger that activates the mudrās is the thumb. The thumb is the fire element, and the fire element (the thumb) activates all the other elements. When we connect the tips of different fingers, it completes a circuit. This circuit then connects all the glands in the body where a particular element is balanced, by either accelerating it or subduing it

Foundational principles of mudrā
Increase or decrease principle

In Mudrās, when we touch the tips of fingers, then we increase or balance the mudrās. When we fold the fingers and press them with the thumb, then we control or decelerate the element.

How does this work?

According to Āyurveda, an imbalance of the elements in the body leads to disease. When this imbalance is corrected at the elemental levels, the gross manifestation of these diseased conditions goes away.

For example, if the earth element is disturbed, then there could be obesity, heaviness, lethargy, etc. in the body. By controlling the earth element, the effects like obesity, etc., can be controlled.

Constitution of our body according to Āyurveda

According to Āyurveda our body is divided into 3 constitutions called kapha, pitta and vāta. The physical structure of our body is called kapha. Kapha is a combination of Earth + Water. All the chemicals and juices like the digestive juices are grouped as pitta. Pitta is a combination of Fire + Water and the transport mechanism in the body is called vāta. Vāta which is a mix of air and ether carries food and oxygen to different parts of the body and removes toxins from the body. Based on the nature and structure of our body Āyurveda divides the body into kapha dominant, pitta dominant and Vāta dominant body.

Here are some key distinguishing features of each type of body. We begin with Vāta

Vāta

1. Body frame is usually thin and does not easily gain weight.
2. Skin dry, rough, dark complexion, cracked.
3. Hair is dry and splits quickly.
4. Quick performance of activities.
5. Variable and/or poor appetite.
6. Less endurance to work for long periods.

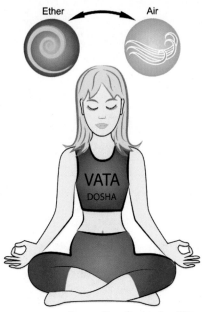

7. Prefers warm or hot food and climate.
8. Scanty perspiration, variable thirst.
9. Tendency to be constipated.
10. Light sleep with many dreams.
11. Very prone to anxiety and therefore they are unpredictable.

Pitta

1. Medium body frame.
2. Skin delicate, warm to touch.
3. Good/excessive appetite.
4. Feels warm/hot sensation.
5. Pitta are heat dominant, so they prefer cooling foods.

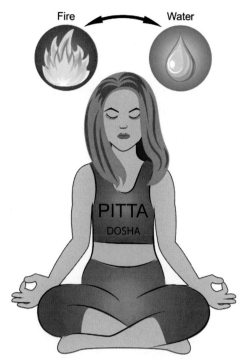

6. Tendency for loose movements.
7. Excessive thirst and perspiration.
8. They have bright eyes and a sharp vision.
9. Hair soft, premature graying, baldness.
10. Hot in temper, brave, intelligent and with good memory.

Kapha

1. Large body frame and easily gain weight.
2. Soft and smooth skin.
3. Good stamina but slow in physical activities.
4. Deep and pleasant voice.

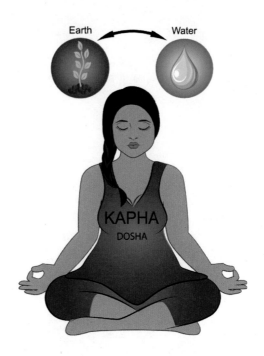

5.   Moderate appetite.

6.   Moderate perspiration, low thirst.

7.   Deep and sound sleep.

8.   Large eyes, calm, stable with whitish sclera.

9.   Hair thick, oily, wavy dark coloured.

10.   Mostly calm.

Balance

The three humors kapha, pitta and vāta must be in balance for good health. Usually, due to heredity and lifestyle, one of the doshas or humors is easily imbalanced. In today's world, hectic lifestyles and use of phones and computers have people shifting their concentration every few seconds, and this has disturbed their eating, sleeping, and lifestyle. When we continuously move from one object to another, the air is the first element disrupted. The other elements follow suit. Remember, Vāta consists of air and ether, disturbance in one element or an Āyurvedic humor also disturbs the other elements.

Mudrās help in balancing

Mudrās balance the elements and Āyurvedic humors. Be it balancing the humor or the elements, mudrās are very beneficial. Certain mudrās like "Musti mudrā" balance all the elements.

Mudrās for the mind

Mind, intelligence and ego are the subtle parts of ourselves according to the yogic scriptures. They are finer than the five elements (earth, water, fire, air and ether). However the mind acts through the five elements. A certain disturbance in the body can create a disturbance in the mind. Similarly when we sit in a meditative position and practice meditative mudrās, it affects the mind in a positive way creating positive thoughts and impressions.

Great yogis in the past like Lord Buddha left behind a series of mudrās by which we can get into deep practices of meditation. By a proper sequence of mudrās which purify our energy channels, energize them and stream positive thoughts, we can achieve whatever we want to achieve in life by proper visualization. These are given in our section -Mudrās for life.

Mudrās for life

At the end of the book you will find a beautiful sequence of mudrās for achieveing different purposes. These sequences are designed to purify the mind, improve our power of intuition, open up the energy channels and let the mind focus on the object or the goal. This series promotes focus, memory and innovation so that we can achieve our purpose. These mudrās can be applied by people of all ages and benefits can be reaped.

In this book the mudrās are presented systematically beginning with the mudrās for five elements;

Mudrās for elements are in the following order

1. Air
    Control with Vāyu mudrā
    Balance with Gyāna mudrā

2. Ether
    Control with Sunya mudrā
    Balance with ākāsha mudrā

3. Earth
    Control with Agni mudrā
    Balance with Prithvi mudrā

4. Water
    Control with Jal Shāmak mudrā
    Balance increase with varuna mudrā

5. Fire: The thumb represents the fire element. According to Āyurveda, most health issues are due to improper digestive heat in the body. The thumb,

which represents fire, is used to increase or decrease all the other elements. So by using the thumb, fire is increased or decreased, which is the core of balancing other elements.

Mudrās for balancing the three humors Kapha, Pitta and vāta

Vāta Balancing - Balancing Air and Ether
Kapha Balancing - Balancing Water and Earth
Pitta Balancing - Balancing Fire and Water

Mudrās for Purification and Memory

In this series we will practice mudrās to purify our nervous systems or Nādis that carry information.By purifying the information highways and their carriers air and ether we can have mental clarity.

Mudrās For Air Element

According to Āyurveda, all diseases in the body and mind are carried and accelerated by an imbalance of the air element. Air is the primary carrier for both physical as well as mental cargo in the body. Of all elements, air needs to be balanced first. When air is balanced, the disease cannot travel far. Even for the healing to begin in the body, the air element needs to be balanced; otherwise, the cure does not take hold. Therefore we begin this book with the essential mudrā for controlling the Vāyu, or air element. This mudrā is called Vāyu mudrā ("that which controls air"). Most diseases today are psychosomatic. Chronic diseases like diabetes, fatigue, and asthma are caused by mental stress leading to improper eating habits, lifestyle, and sleep. All bad habits lead to an imbalance in air within our bodies.

Benefits of Vayu (air) Mudrās: Air controlling and balancing mudrās must be practiced before most other mudrās. Once air is balanced, other elements can be balanced and benefits can be derived.

We start with the air control mudrā, or the Vāyu mudrā.

Vāyu Mudrā

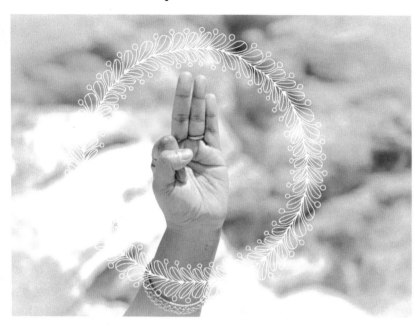

Method - Fold the forefinger of each hand to touch the base of each thumb. Now cover the forefingers with the thumbs as shown.

For all therapeutic (chronic disease healing) purposes, mudrās, including this one, should be held for 40 minutes or more. The more concentrated we hold it, the better the effect.

Benefits - Calms the air pressure in the body and mind, reducing anxiety which in turn is the base for other elements to be controlled. Balances hormonal flow, clears voice and mind.

Special healing properties

This mudrā is very beneficial in problems relating to knee pain, rheumatism and joint related problems like arthritis, paralysis including facial paralysis.
Regular practice of this mudra can reduce the effect of parkinsons disease. Another very effective area is for stiff neck.

Astrologically Vāyu mudrā is useful for Saturn lines on the hand (Saturn causes gas). Vāyu mudrā should be practiced along with Prāṇa mudrā for better benefits.

Practice sequence for Vayu Mudrā

1. Sit in a comfortable position.
2. Join the hands at the top of your head.
3. Praying to the universal energy connect to the life of the universe. Keep back straight.
4. Now fold the forefinger and cover it with the thumb. Touch the tip of the forefinger to the base of the thumb.
5. Focus on the thumb and the tip of the forefinger touching the palm.
6. Focus your attention on the touch to the palm. This actuates the pituitary gland and all the primary functions of the brain by energizing the neurons.
7. Keep focussing on the mudrā for 10-20 minutes.
8. Now practice Prāṇa mudrā (52) for 10 minutes.
9. Join your hands and end with a prayer.

Gyāna Mudrā (Air Balancer)

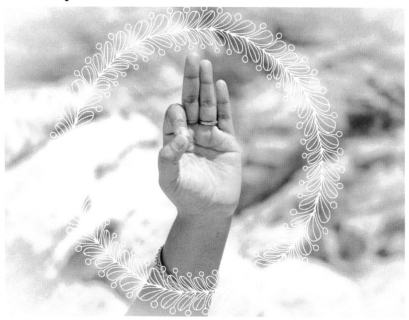

Method: Join the tips of your Index Finger and thumb to form the Gyān mudrā.

Benefits

Improves memory and concentration. Gyāna mudrā is used in all sitting meditative poses. Depression, lack of enthusiasm, and lack of clarity can be addressed with Gyāna mudrā. It is also called Abhay Gyāna mudrā, Vāyu Vardhak mudrā, Purna Gyāna mudrā. This mudrā heals insomnia and cures lunacy.

Q. When and how long do we practice Gyāna Mudrā?

Gyāna Mudrā can be practiced as long as you can. The longer you practice the better the results you get. You can practice it while walking and sitting. However when you practice it in a very concentrated manner you will get better results especially sitting in Padmāsana or Siddhāsana.

What are the subtle points of practice in Gyāna Mudrā

When we touch the tips of the thumb and the forefinger gently we can feel the pulse. If we concentrate on the pulse, we will feel a healing energy in the body and in between the eyebrows (the third eye). When we fully focus on this pulse, we activate the neurons in the brain and we feel calm and focused.

How to practice Gyāna Mudrā

1. Sit in a comfortable position.
2. Join the hands in namaste position at the top of your head.
3. Praying to the universal energy connect to all the elements in the universe. Keep back straight.
4. Bring the hands in front of your chest and hold them in a prayer position.
5. Keep the hands on both your knees with fingers pointing upwards.
6. Now touch the tips of the fore fingers and the thumb. As you touch them, the touch should be gentle, and you will feel

the pulse.

7. As soon as you feel the pulse, concentrate on the pulse.
8. This actuates the pituitary gland and all the primary functions of the brain by energizing the neurons.
9. Keep focussing on the mudrā.
10. Focus on your breath and the pulse.
11. Fully immerse your mind only in the breathing and the pulse.
12. Practise anywhere between 15 - 45 minutes and you will get very good results. Longer duration of practice yiled better results.

Note : This sequence applies to other mudrās as well. Any mudra should be practiced for a minimum of 15 minutes. Some mudrās like Gyāna mudrās can be practiced for any length of time. For each mudrās we will designate how long we can practice them.

Mudrās for Ether element

Ether is the element that contains sound. In Sanskrit it is called ākāsha, or space. Our bodies and minds have limited spaces. With the amount of radiation we are exposed to due to the electronic gadgets we use, we fill our available ethereal space with so much sound that it overwhelms the system, and we cannot think or act clearly. A common saying goes when we are overwhelmed "Give me my space". We need to balance these sounds, clear up the ethereal speace for a better train of thought. A combination of air and ether is the Vāta humor in Āyurveda. If one or the other is imbalanced, then Vāta is imbalanced.

When space or ākāsha is disturbed, it impairs our hearing and our ability to comprehend. Problems like tinnitus tend to surface. A yogi heals by hearing calming sounds like that of birds chirping, sound of flowing river, soft breeze, kirtans, healing instrumental music, and mudrā practice.

Other important aspects of Ether principle

The ether principle is related to strength in the bones and the heart. When the ether principle is active, our bones get stronger; otherwise, the bones feel lifeless and weak.
The middle finger, which represents the sky element, is related to the heart. The heart functions efficiently by the constant practice of this mudra. Ether mudras also improve the production of blood. Blood is produced from bone marow, and ether mudras help enhance the quality of blood.

Decelarating space : Śūnya mudrā

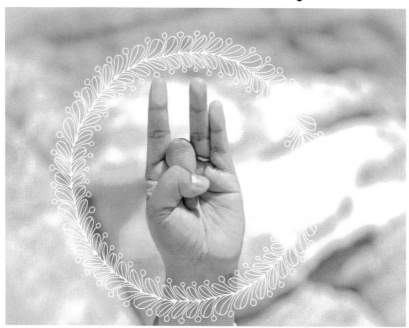

Method - Fold the middle finger as shown and touch the tip of the middle finger to the base of the thumb. Cover the finger with the thumb as shown.

Benefits - Ether is one of the components of vāta in the body. Hearing, thinking and focus depend on air and ether. When we are stressed, air and ether accelerate, leading to uncontrolled thoughts which result in a host of problems such as loss of hearing. By this mudrā, all issues relating to ether can be controlled and healed.

Ears : This mudrā benefits the ears by healing the hearing loss and improving the clarity of hearing.

33

The mudrā related to ether unlike the mudras related to air should be practiced for certain periods of time only.

Practice sequence for Sūnya Mudrā

1. Sit in a comfortable position.
2. Join the hands at the top of your head.
3. Praying to the universal energy, connect to the life of the universe. Keep your back straight. Bring hands down and keep the hands on on your knees or just above.
4. Now fold the middle finger and cover it with the thumb. Touch the tip of the middle finger and the base of the thumb.
5. Focus on the thumb and the tip of the middle finger touching the palm.
6. Focus your attention on the touch sensation of the middle finger and the palm. This actuates the heart and all the primary functions of the heart by opening the space of thoughts that clog the heart and also the ears.
7. Keep focussing on the mudrā for 10-25 minutes.
8. Now practice Prāṇa mudrā for 10 minutes.
9. Join your hands and end with a prayer.

Do not perform this mudrā for long periods of time.

Balancing space : Ākāsha mudrā

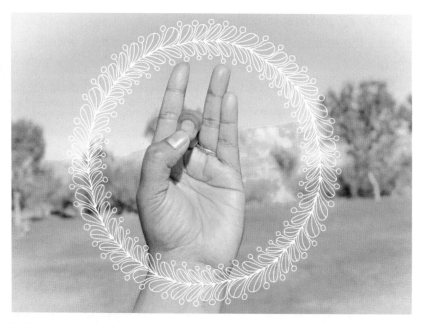

Method : Gently touch the tip of middle finger and the thumb. Feel the pulse.

Benefits: This mudra increases space. It is considered to augment meditation and focus. Space, or ether, holds sound (connected to thought and hearing).

As in the previous mudrā, this mudrā also improves the hearing by increasing and balancing space. This space also improves production of sound. It also improves the heart space. The flow of prāṇa and consequently the flow of blood in the heart region can be done by this mudrā.

1. Sit in a comfortable position.
2. Join the hands in namaste position at the top of your head.
3. Praying to the universal energy connect to all the elements in the universe. Keep back straight.
4. Bring the hands in front of your chest and hold them in a prayer position.
5. Keep the hands on both your knees with fingers pointing upwards.
6. Now touch the tips of the forefinger and the middle fingers. As you touch them, the touch should be gentle, and you will feel the pulse.
7. As soon as you feel the pulse, concentrate on the pulse.
8. Focus your attention on the pulse. This actuates the Heart chakra and energizes the ether or the space element in the body.
9. Keep focussing on the mudrā.
10. Focus on your breath and the pulse.
11. Immerse your mind in the breathing and the pulse sensation.
12. Practise anywhere between 15 - 25 minutes and you will get very good results.

Mudrās for Earth element

Prithvi, or earth element, is a combination of all elements. Hence it deals with the whole body, particularly the body weight. The earth element dominates muscles, bones, tendons, and all other organs in the body. Therefore the earth element can be used to increase or decrease body weight. Heaviness is a characteristic resulting from the earth element being disturbed. Prithvi also controls the sense of smell and even the texture of the skin.

The earth principle governs all the "previous" elements of sound, sight, taste, and smell. This mudrā activates and helps them function entirely. Here "previous" means referring to the origin of creation (according to yogic scriptures), we find that the first element created is ether, ether transforms to air, air to fire, fire condenses to water and all of them combine to form earth. The next element consists of the previous element in the cycle.

Controlling Earth : Sūrya mudrā

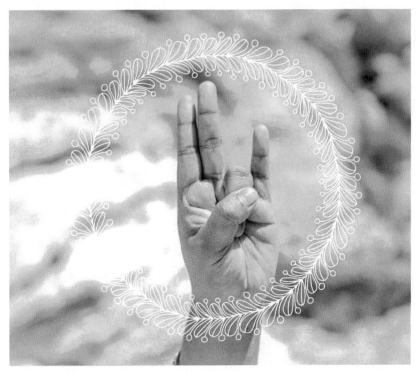

Sūrya mudrā increases the fire element and decreases the earth element in the body. The fire element is related to vision, improving fire in the body, clears visual problems. Since agni (fire) is the main component of pitta humor, this mudrā improves pitta, enhancing digestion, and reducing fat in the body leading to weight control. For all constipation related issues, Sūrya mudrā is the best.

Useful for skin ailments and improves blood circulation. It helps us stay grounded as well.

Herein thumb (the symbol of fire principle) presses the ring finger (the earth principle). The earth principle is responsible for the growth of muscles which is hindered by extra fat. this fat begins to melt with Sūrya mudrā.

Highlights : When the ring finger and thumb are pressed properly the pineal and pituitary glands are activated. The thyroid and parathyroid glands are also activated leading to a great improvement in digestion.

Practicing sūrya mudrā for just 10 - 20 minutes a day will help reduce fat in the body. This mudrā is beneficial for asthma, cold, digestion, sinus, TB and pneumonia.

Mudrā practice for weight loss

1. Sit in a comfortable position.
2. Join the hands in namaste position at the top of your head.
3. Praying to the universal energy connect to all the elements in the universe. Keep back straight.
4. Bring the hands in front of your chest and hold them in a prayer position.
6. This actuates the pineal, pituitary, thyroid and parathyroid glands
7. Focus on the middle of the eyebrows and feel the energy at that point. You will feel an increase of heat in the body. Meditate on fire of digestion in the belly. Meditate on the manipura chakra(navel).

7. Keep focussing on the Sūrya mudrā for 10-20 minutes.

8. Now practice Jal Shāmak mudra(44) for 10 minutes.

9. Now practice Linga Mudrā for 10 minutes.

10. Thank the healing energy for healing body, mind and skin.

11. Join your hands and end with a prayer.

Balancing Earth : Prithvi mudrā

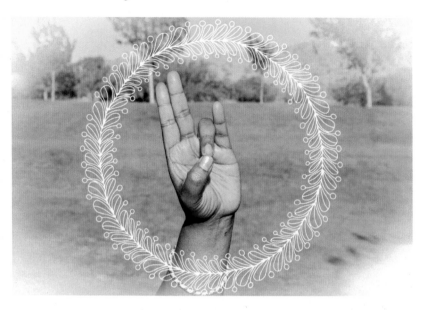

Method: Touch the tip of the ring finger and the thumb. Earth is a significant component of our bodily organs. The practice of Prithvi mudrā strengthens all the organs.

Benefits : Prithvi mudrā gives strength to the muscles and bones. It reduces the burning sensation in the body by reducing the fire element and improving the earth element. It is very useful for hyperthyroidism.

BMI index is balanced. Improves skin radiance as skin is related to the earth element. Balancing the earth element balances all the elements and brings about a sense of fulfillment.

Earth element is related to the root chakra and balancing the earth element helps us stay grounded.

Since it improves the earth element it also helps heals asthma.

Balancing Fire Element

Mudrās for water element

Our bodies are 80% water. Water facilitates the flow of fluids in the body. We need water at an optimum temperature and at the right viscosity for a proper flow. Water element is a component of both kapha and pitta elements. A disturbance in water component creates a disturbance in both kapha and pitta. The two primary mudrās to increase and decrease the water element are dealt within this section along with their benefits.

Controlling Water: Jal Shāmak Mudrā

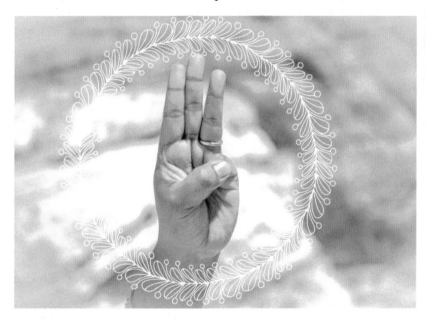

Method: Fold the little finger so that its tip touches the base of the thumb. Cover the little finger with the thumb as shown.

Benefits : This mudrā decreases the water element, which is the main component of Kapha humor. When water is pressed by the fire principle, it reduces the excess water content.

Hence diseases caused by Kapha elements like runny nose, sinus, excess salivation, throat pain, bad cold, excess urination, bedwetting, obesity and watery eyes can be gradually controlled by this mudrā. Hyperacidity, diarrhea can also be treated with the practice of this mudrā.

Practicing for 45 minutes everyday will let excess fat gets dissolved in ones body. This mudrā should be practiced along with the sūrya mudra in the weight loss sequence.

For reducing the water content in the body practice Jal Shāmak Mudrā in the same sequence as vāyu mudra replacing the vāyu mudra with Jal Shāmak mudrā.

Balancing water : Varuṇa Mudrā

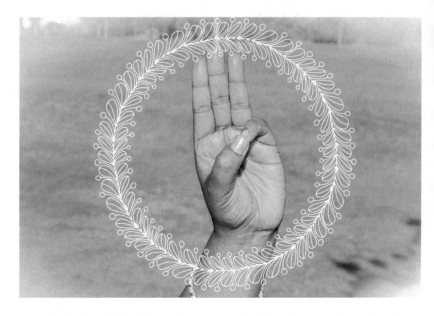

Method: Fold the little finger so that its tip touches the tip of the thumb. Touch softly and feel the pulse.

Benefits: Varuṇa mudrā increases and balances the water element in the body. Water is present in all bodily juices such as lymph, blood, tears, saliva, mucus, digestive juices, enzymes, hormones, semen, cerebrospinal fluid, etc. This mudrā keeps them properly hydrated so that their functioning is smooth. It keeps the mouth moist, and the secretion of saliva is balanced, which improves the sense of taste and digest the food. According to Āyurveda, our digestion improves when the taste buds are fully active. Cramps and dehydration can also be treated effectively.

Note : Varuṇa mudrā should be practiced when it is needed for a limited time only (Its meant mainly for healing ailments, until the ailment exists).

The problems caused due to lack of water or dryness are overcome by Varuṇa mudrā. It keeps the skin fresh and prevents the diseases of the skin. It is a panacea for dry cough.

Varuṇa mudrā is especially helpful in the summer, when due to heat we may feel dehydrated and develop related problems.

Vāta, Pitta and Kapha

Stress results in too many thoughts. Long term stress results in uncontrolled airflow and ringing sounds in the ears. This is due excess vāta which is a combination of air and ether. Excess Vāta also magnifies the impact of all other diseases. Hence we control Vāta by using the two fingers representing vāta, the forefinger, and the middle finger.

Similarly when earth and water are imbalanced together, then that is called kapha imbalance and we need to apply the fingers pertaining to earth and water together to balance kapha

Finally pitta which is a combination of fire and water needs to be balanced as pitta aggravation leads to acidity, heartburn, etc. But the way to control pitta is by increasing or decreasing kapha. By increasing kapha we decrease pitta and by decreasing kapha we increase pitta.

We can also work on two humors at once like vāta and kapha by using the fingers related to the humors.

Vāta-Nāshak Mudrā

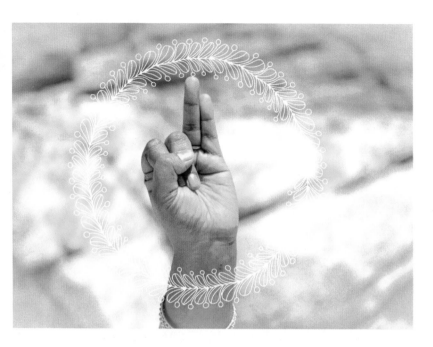

Method: Fold the forefinger and the middle finger, touching their tips to the base of the thumb. Now press the fingers with the thumb, as shown.

Benefits: Vāta-nāshak mudrā helps overcome indecisiveness, impatience, hyperactivity by calming you down. The calming effect can put you to good sleep. Effective on insomnia as it calms the mind. Issues like giddiness, vertigo, joint pains, Parkinson's disease can also be treated with this mudrā.

Increasing Vāta : Vāyān Mudrā

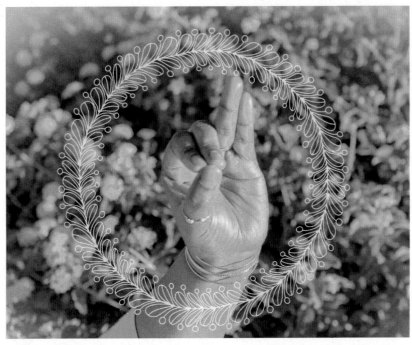

Method: Gently touch the tips of the forefinger and middle fingers to the tip of the thumb.

Benefits: When Vāta is deficient, it can result in the another set of problems like depression, slowness of body, and mind. In this case, we have to increase the Vāta by touching the forefinger and middle fingertips with the thumb.

Vāyān mudrā overcomes nervous exhaustion and nervous breakdown, lifts our spirit, enthusiasm and optimism by balancing Vāta (a combination of air and ether which are the carriers of sound and energy in the body and the mind).

Controlling Kapha (Increase Pitta)

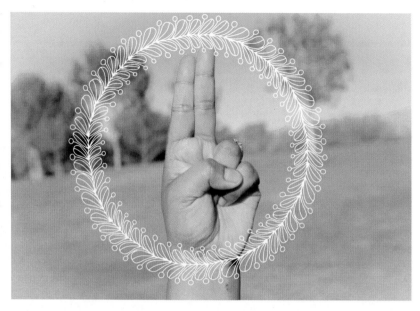

Kapha-nāshak mudrā decreases kapha humor and increases pitta humor. Pitta plays a significant role in the heat and digestion of the body. This mudrā is good for those who have a deficiency in pitta and have excess Kapha.

Benefits and healing properties

With increased heat, energy levels increase, lethargy goes down. In the winter season it heats the body and improves digestion. Kapha is responsible for the wet (excess phlegm) and a greasy body. By controlling kapha (when it is in excess), problems of oily skin and excess phlegm goes away. This, in turn, improves the respiratory system.

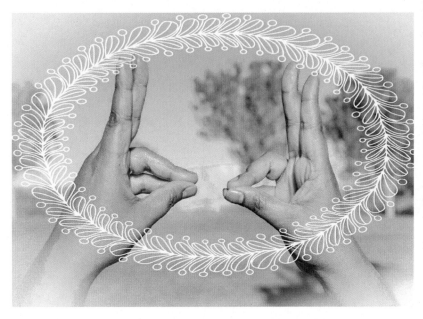

Prāṇa mudrā increases kapha humor, which is responsible for body structure, energy levels and immunity.

Method: Join the tips of the ring finger, little finger, and the thumb. This will form Prāṇa mudrā.

Benefits: Prāṇa mudrā is instrumental in the treatments of chronic fatigue, general debility, low endurance, impaired immunity, mental tension, anger and irritability. Some of the other issues where this mudrā is useful are hyperthyroidism, inflammatory disorders, ulcers, arthritis, etc.

Prāṇa mudrā activates the various energy centers in the body. It acts like a dynamo. It also increases the life energy.

According to astrology ring finger represents the sun principle. Sun is responsible for giving us heat and light. The little finger stands for mercury which is responsible for the water element. When earth, water and fire come together they form a powerful combination of energy flow.

This mudrā effectively increases the circulation of blood resulting in strengthening of muscles and improvement in vision.

For insomnia

Prāṇa mudrā when practiced with Gyāna mudrā cures insomnia.

For Diabetes

When Prāṇa mudrā is practiced with Apāṇa mudrā, Apāṇa Vāyu mudrā , and Samana mudrā diabetes can be controlled.

Sequence for Insomnia

1. Laydown in a comfortable position.
2. Practice Gyāna mudrā.
3. Focus on your breath and the pulse.
4. Practise for 20 minutes
5. Close your eyes, calm down and relax.

6. Now practice Prāṇa mudrā for 20 minutes.

7. Throughout the practice let go of all other thoughts and simply focus on your breath and feel the difference.

Sequence for Diabetes

1. Sit in a comfortable position.

2. Join the hands at the top of your head.

3. Praying to the universal energy connect to the universal elements. Keep back straight.

4. Practice Apāna mudrā. When you touch the tips of the fingers keep focussing on the pulse. (15 minutes)

5. Practice Apāṇa Vāyu mudrā (15 minutes)

6. Practice Sāmana Vāyu mudrā for 15 minutes.

7. Now practice Prāṇa mudrā for 10 minutes.

8. Join your hands and end with a soothing prayer.

Vāta Kapha Nāshaka

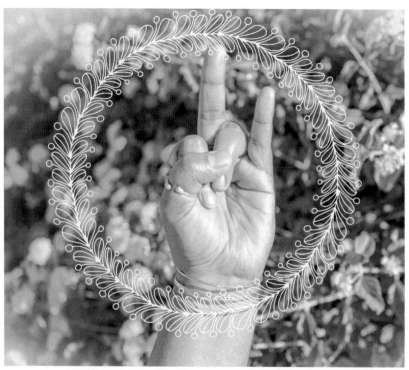

This mudrā balances vāta+kapha healing ailments, which are caused by a combination of both Vāta and Kapha.

Method: Touch the tips of forefinger and ring fingers to the base of the thumb and cover the fingers with the thumb, as shown.

Duration: 45 minutes every day, either at one stretch or in three parts (i.e., for 15 minutes, thrice a day)

Vāta Pitta Nāshaka

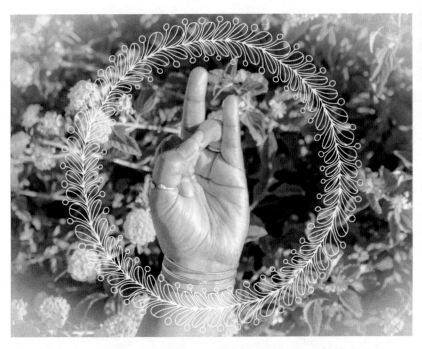

As the name suggests, Vāta and pitta nāshak mudrā helps overcome both Vāta and pitta imbalance issues.

Method: Place the tip of the index finger at the base of the thumb and gently touch the tip of the ring finger with the tip of the thumb.

One who is kapha dominant should practice this mudrā in moderation only.

Tridosha Balancer - Surabhi

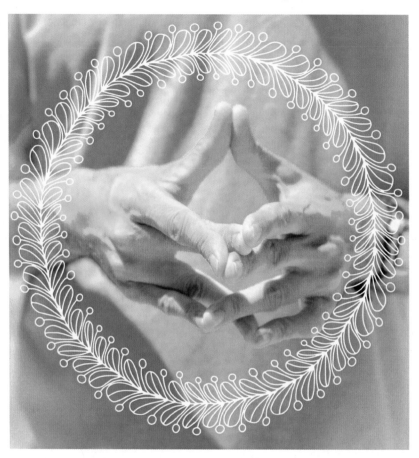

Surabhi Mudrā : Surabhi mudrā controls the adverse effects of all three doshas or humors. It also balances all five elements in the body. Surabhi means cow, and the cow is sacred in the Vedic paradigm, one who fulfills all desires, so does this mudrā.

Method: Step 1. Cross the forefinger and middle finger of your right hand. Similarly cross the little finger and ring finger of the right hand.

Step 2. Left hand: Gently touch the left hand forefinger's tip to the middle finger of the right hand and middle finger of the left to the forefinger of the right.

Step 3. Similarly, touch the tip of the ring finger of the left hand to the little finger of the right hand and the tip of the left-hand little finger of the left hand to the ring finger of the right hand.

Benefits : When practiced regulary this mudrā balances all the three humors Kapha, Pitta and Vāta

Pañcha Vāyus (Five Airs)

The next most important concept is that of five airs or pañcha vāyus. As mentioend earlier air is the main carrier of energy and thoughts in the body.

The movements of the body are first generated from the heart, and all the activities of the body are made possible by the senses, powered by the five kinds of air within the body.

The main air passing through the nose in breathing is called Prāṇa. The air which passes through the rectum as evacuated bodily air is called apāna. The air which adjusts and digests the foodstuff within the stomach and which sometimes sounds as belching is called samāna. The air which passes through the throat and the stoppage of which constitutes suffocation is called the udāna air. And the total air which circulates throughout the entire body is called the vyāna air.

Prāṇa Mudrā

Prāṇa air is responsible for the upward movement of air and energy. When *prāṇa* is low we feel weak. The mudrā pertaining to the *prāṇa* air is *prāṇa* mudrā. (See page 52) By performing this mudrā we increase energy levels in the body.

Vyāna Vāyu Mudrā

Please read the Vāyān mudrā (See page 50) . Every organ in our body is situated in space and held in its place by the pressure of air. This pressure of air which pervades the whole body balancing it is called Vyāna air. Vāyān Mudrā balances this air.

Apāna Mudrā

Excess or lack of perspiration, excess or lack of urine and stool causes disease. The air in the lower part of the body pushing the waste down is called apāna vāyu. There are two mudrās which help the downward movement of air, apāna mudrā and apāna vāyu mudrā.

These two mudrās heal excess gas, prostrate gland problems and in general problems related to all excretory organs. Fistlua and hemorrhoids can be avoided by the practice of apāna mudrā.

Apāna vāyu is very beneficial for healing diabetes as it helps eliminate the toxins. The sequence for diabetes has already been described before in page 54. Expectant mothers can also perform this mudrā in the last month of pregnancy.

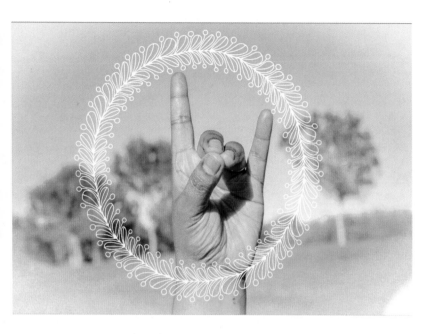

Apāna vāyu deals with the downward movement of toxins in the body, namely stool, and urine. When this air is not functioning correctly, we can experience constipation, indgestion, etc.

Apāna mudrā, which is a combination of Prithvi (earth) and Ākāsh (ether) mudrā, improves the Apāna vāyu, thereby leading to proper elimination of waste.

Apāna Vāyu Mudrā

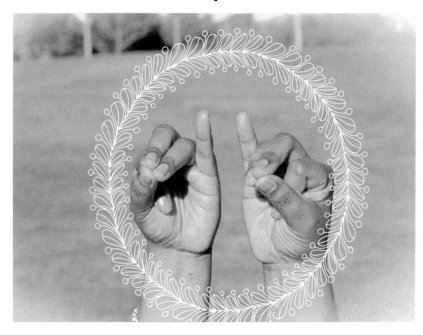

Method : Fold the forefinger and touch the tip to the base of the thumb, now gently touch the tip of thumb, middle finger and the ring finger.

Benefits : This mudrā increases circulation by thinning the blood. This is also called heart mudrā as it revitalizes the heart, removes blockages and improving circulation. Therefore this mudra is called Hridaya (heart) mudrā.

This mudrā can work effectively to prevent symptoms of heart attack. It relives the stomach of excess gas which in turn helps the heart.

Pressure , tiredness and excess perspiration are all the symptons of a heart attack. Start practicing this mudrā as soon as you notice these symptoms.

This mudrā heals tensions, tiredness, blocks in the blood veins. Also removes cholesterol to a greater degree.

Samana Vāyu Mudrā

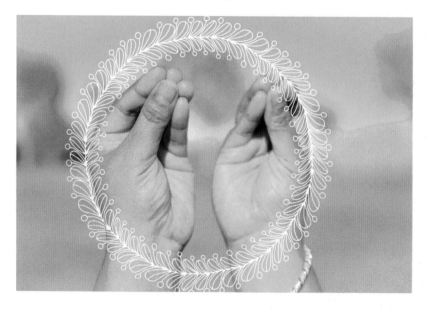

Samana Vāyu Mudrā deals with the fire of digestion in the stomach. It's the primary source of heat and energy in the body. The samāna mudrā improves this agni and our digestive power.

When we meditate on the fingers' tips by gently touching all the tips together, it creates beautiful energy of healing. We can place these fingers on different parts of the body that need healing akin to reiki. Meditation has been added later based on this healing mechanism.

This is a very important mudrā to balance all the elements and can be practiced any time as long as we can.

Udana Vāyu Mudrā

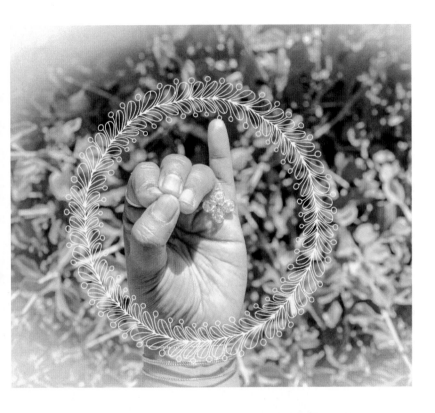

Udana vāyu, or "ascending air," is the vāyu that directs energy from lower to upper chakras. It lies between the heart and the head. Udana vāyu balances the pressure in the head and the body. The loudness and clarity of communication from the throat and our ability to float while swimming depends on Udana vāyu.

Method : Gently touch the the tips of all the fingers except the little finger as shown.

Mudrās for Improving heat/digestion

Musti Mudrā

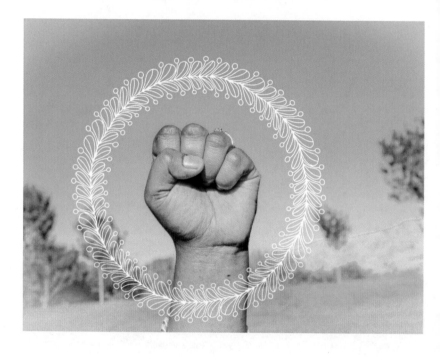

Musti is a sanskrit word meaning closed hand or fist. When we are emotionally charged, we clench our fists to release emotions. This clenching of the fist is also a mudrā that can effectively improve our digestive levels. Closing all fingers and covering them with the thumb is called Musti mudrā. After lunch, if we take a walk with this mudrā, our digestion improves.

Ādi Mudrā

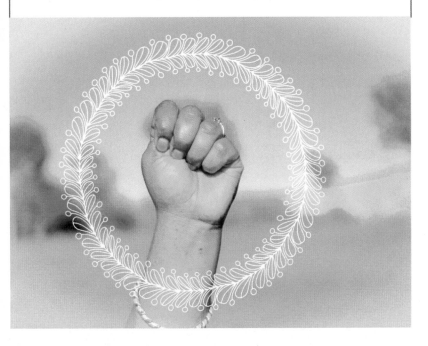

This is similar to the previous mudrā. However the difference is that the thumb covered by all the other fingers as shown.

This mudrā helps release all emotions which are pent up in our heart and calms us after sometime. Ādi mudrā is practiced when emotions are high. When practiced with deep breathing it has a tremendous effect and calms down emotions.

Linga Mudrā

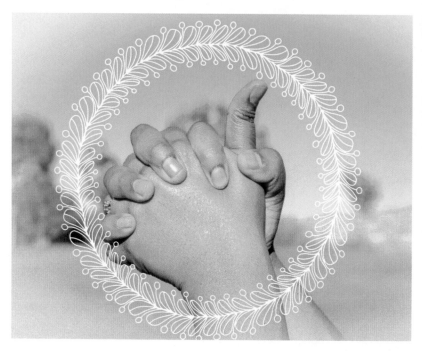

Method : Clasp both the hands and lift the thumb of the left hand as shown.

Benefits : This mudrā increases heat levels in the body. It increases circulation and improves digestion.

In the winter season linga mudrā heats up the body. Those with chronic pitta must avoid this mudrā. Regular practice of linga mudrā activates thyroid, parathyroid glands, liver and pancreas due to heat. Heals neck pain and diseases associated with cold.

Pūshan Mudrā

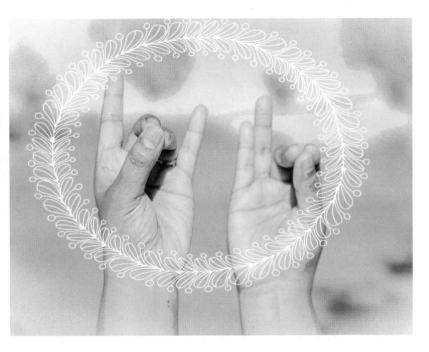

Method : On the left hand gently touch the tips of middle finger, ring finger and the thumb. Simultaneously on the right hand gently touch the thumb, forefinger and the middle finger.

Benefits : This mudrā increases heat leavels in the body, increases circulation and improves digestion.

Meditative Mudrās

Mudrās can be applied for several purposes. Healing, strengthening, and meditating. So far, we have come to understand healing mudrās. Now we will understand meditative mudrās. Meditation means one-pointedness of the mind. This concentration of the mind is the function of the air; therefore, the Gyāna mudrā is the most commonly used mudrā for meditation. Lord Buddha has felt behind several mudrās for meditation. His mudrā sequences help us achieve peace, calmness and clarity of mind. We have dealt with those powerful mudrās given by Lord Buddha in this book.

Meditation begins with purification. This purification can be achieved by two special mudrās. Śaṅkha mudrā and Sahaj Śaṅkha mudrā. If we hold these mudrās between five to ten minutes, accompanied by a deep breath, all the seventy-two thousand nerves are purified.

By purifying the nerves, Śaṅkha mudrā relieves stress, tension, negative emotions, negative thoughts, and sets the ground for meditation. Therefore Śaṅkha mudrā is practiced at the very beginning. And this lays the ground where other meditative mudrās become very effective.

The Sahaja Śaṅkha mudrā is a more relaxed version of the Śaṅkha mudrā. The Sahaja Śaṅkha mudrā gives a similar effect as the Śaṅkha mudrā but also activates the Manipura chakra improving digestion of the food in the stomach and digestion of thoughts in the mind.

Śaṅkha Mudrā

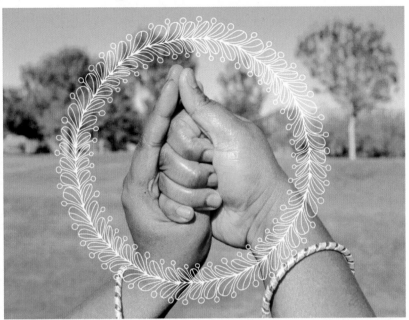

Method : Open up the left hand,. Then clasp the left hand's thumb with the first four fingers of the right hand and gently touch the thumb of the right hand with the forefinger and the middle finger of the left hand as shown.

Benefits : Śaṅkha or conch has much to do with sound and purification. In Vedic tradition, conch is considered pure, and the sound emanating from the conch is very purifying, driving away fears and improving confidence. Similarly, this mudrā purifies all the 72,000 nādis (subtle nerves) and enhances the flow of thought and memory retention. This, in turn, leads to better memory, soothing of the mind. Before any mantra chanting, practicing this mudrā is recommended.

This mudrā is known to keep our voice in good condition as it influences the thyroid and the throat muscles. One gains a sweet voice and overcomes stammering if one has any.

This mudrā purifies all the 72,000 nadis (subtle nerves) in the body. These subtle nadis carry thoughts and energy within the body.

The Śaṅkha mudrā also activates Manipura chakra thereby curing the ailments of stomach and interstine. Kidneys are purified by this mudrā. It also heals tonsils and acts as an anti-dote to dust allergy. People suffering from mouth ulcers can be cured effectively.

In the practice of mudrās for detox, Śaṅkha mudrā is the first mudrā.

Sahaj Śaṅkha Mudrā

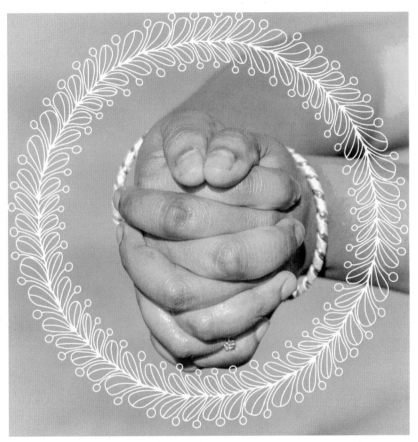

Sahaj means easy, and the Sahaj Śaṅkha mudrā is an easier version of the Śaṅkha mudrā. Its very easy to perform compared to the Śaṅkha mudrā. This will give you almost similar results, however some yogis consider it even better.

Clasp both hands and interlock all the fingers as shown and hold the thumbs straight as shown. This can be performed in place of or in conjunction with Śaṅkha mudrā.

At the base of the thumb, the soft fleshy part is connected to the manipura chakra and the stomach. This mudrā along with the Śaṅkha mudrā activates the base of the thumb which is connected to the Manipura chakra (the fire chakra).

All the major nerves of the body are purified by the practice of this mudrā. Digestion improves, bodily strength increases, Gastric problems and hemorrhoids are healed.

Ganesha Mudrā

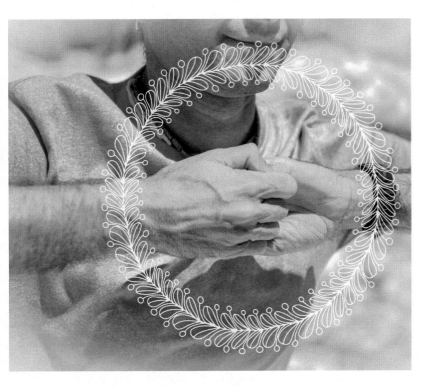

Method : Bring both hands near the chest. Bend your fingers and form a "U" with all fingers. Now slide your hands into each other so that the fingers lock into each other. Hold them not too tight or loose. Hold them comfortably.

Benefits : This mudrā when done with the rememberance of Lord Ganesha removes all obstacles. Vows can be taken in this mudrā as the power of Ganesha makes the vow successful. Apply this mudrā before you take any vow of meditation or healing.

Rudra Mudrā

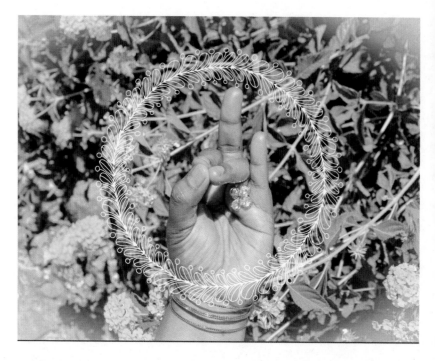

Method : Gently touch the tips of the thumb, forefinger, and ring finger, as shown.

Benefits : This mudrā improves circulation, respiration, and energizes the body, improving memory and mental clarity. Very beneficial for those who have issues with depression.

Dharmachakra Mudrā

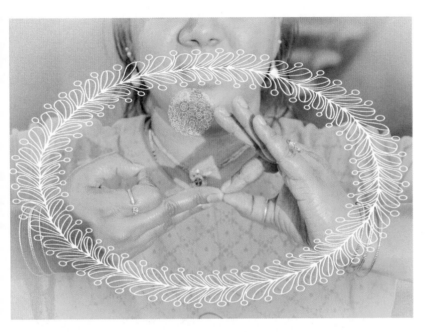

Method : Gently touch together the tips of the thumb and forefinger of the right hand. Now gently touch the tips of thumb and forefinger of the left hand, and gently touch these two fingers (of the left hand) to the tips of the middle finger of the right hand, as shown. Hold the hands at the level of the heart during this mudrā.

Benefits : This mudrā calms the mind and streamlines the thoughts. It balances both sides of the brain and the mind. This mudrā will be used in the meditation sequence at the end of the book.

Karana Mudrā

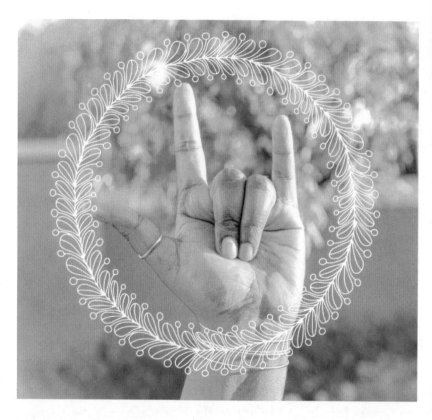

Method : Fold the middle finger and ring finger and touch their tips to the palm as shown.

Benefits : This mudrā is practiced as a part of the Buddhist meditation sequence to expel negative energies. All those forces that block our progress are expelled.

Ksepana Mudrā

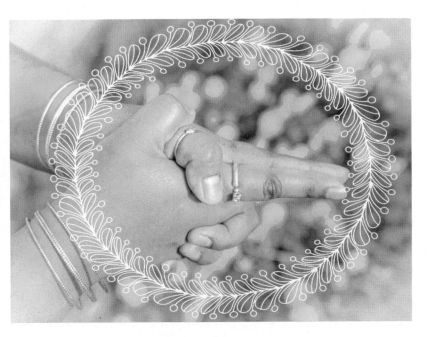

Method: Clasp fingers of both the hands, only extending the forefingers as shown.

Benefits: This mudrā is practiced as a part of the Buddhist meditation sequence. This mudrā fills up the body and mind with nectar or very powerful energy. We will apply this mudrā as a part of meditation to improve energy levels in the body and mind.

Ksepana mudra also detoxes the body. It strengthens the large interstines, lungs and skin.

Dhyāna Mudrā

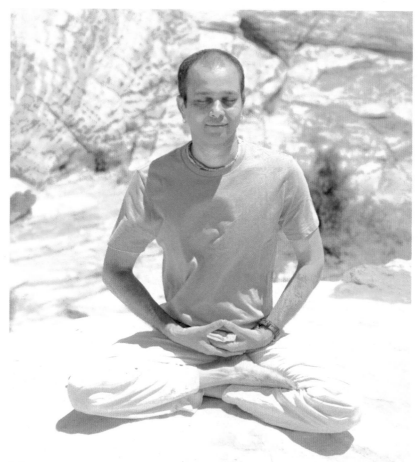

Method: Sit in any comfortable sitting posture with back straight. Place the palm of one hand on the other and touch the thumbs as shown. You can change the hands at every meditation.

Benefits: This mudrā improves the level of concentration of the mind. It is practiced for achieving deeper levels of meditation.

Gyāna Mudrā

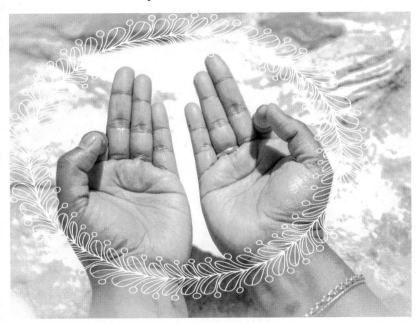

Method: Gently touch the tips of forefingers and the thumb in both hands. If you gently touch the tips you will feel the pulse. This mudrā is the best for meditation , concentration and memory.

Mudrā for Memory

Memory and clarity of thought are the functions of the mind. The mind is connected via a subtle set of nerves to the various organs of the body. These connections pass via the chakras and the glands, which act as transmitters for different bodily energies. When the channels carrying these energies and thoughts are cleansed, our memory improves. In other words, the mind becomes aware of the thoughts within these energy channels. The Gyāna or the air balancing mudrā is one of the best mudrās to improve our memory. Gyāna and Hākini mudrās are considered best for memory.

Mudrā for Memory : Hākini Mudrā

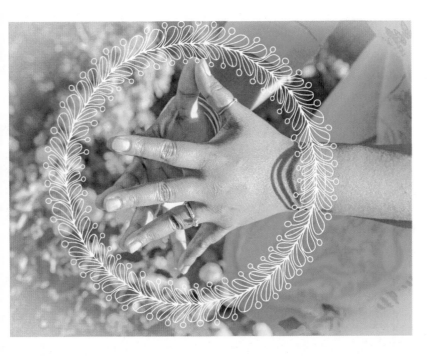

Method: Bring both hands close together and gradually touch the tips of respective fingers, as shown. Feel the pulse at the tip of each finger. Hold for about 20 minutes.

Benefits: Hākini mudrā enhances memory. Used in many corporate environments, this mudrā is known to help remember minute details of meetings and talks. When practiced, this mudrā rewires both sides of the brain giving the desired effect

Mudrā for Detox

Beginning with along with Makara mudrā, we will now look at a series of mudrās to detox and heal the body. Our excretory and digestive systems carry a lot of toxins which needs to cleaned periodically. If toxins not cleaned, then they can build up and cause disease. After cleansing, we rejuvinate the body with Prāṇa mudrā.

After all the mudrās are presented we have put them in a series in which to practice.

You can practice this series along with us on our website

www.yoginataraj.com/mudra

Makara Mudrā

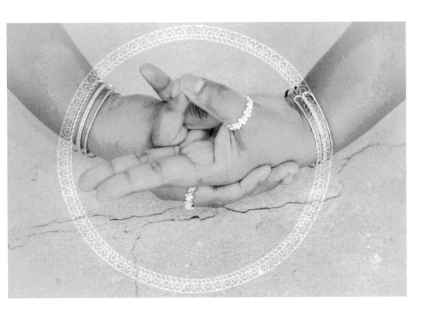

Place left hand on the right, insert the right thumb, between the left small and ring fingers, and place it at the center of the left hand. Touch the left ring finger with the tip of the left thumb. With the remaining fingers hold the hands.

Benefits: Activates the kidneys. Clears up the dark circles around the eyes caused by weakness. Prāṇa mudrā, along with the Makara mudrā, can get the desired result quicker. 20-25 minutes.

Matangi Mudrā

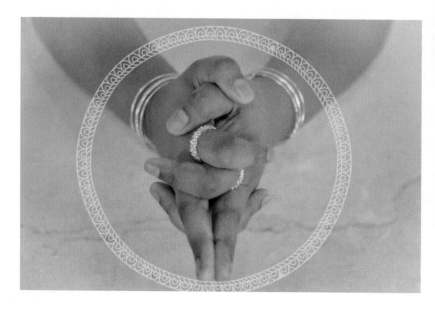

Stretch the middle fingers of both hands representing ether element. Let them touch each other, When you touch the top of the fingers firmly (not too hard) you will feel the pulse. Let other fingers remain interlocked, as shown in the figure. Place the left thumb over the right thumb.

Benefits: This mudrā activates the earth and space principle in the body. It makes one's heart, liver, and kidneys, duodenum, and gall bladder stronger.

Yoni Mudra

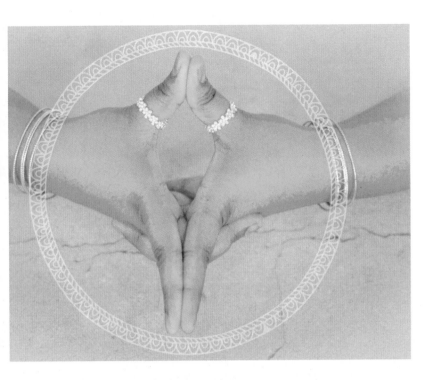

Join the thumbs of both hands (which symbolize Agni (fire principle)) and index fingers (representing the vayu principle). Interlock the other fingers. The thumbs will be facing upwards, and the index fingers will be facing downwards. This vinyasa is called the Yoni mudrā.

This mudrā is specially designed for women. The vinyasa of yoni mudra is kept below the stomach pelvis (yoni).

Special features

As thumbs and index fingers touch each other, they generate an immense volume of heat and vibrations of these elements. As the fingers remain interlocked, they solve several problems related to the womb and the pelvic region.

Benefits

Yoni mudra is very beneficial for women during menstrual cycle. The mudrā must be done in isolation (being alone in the room). After sometime *Prāṇa* mudra must be done for 10- 15 minutes in the morning. Once the mestrual cycle is normal then this mudrā practice must be stopped. After the age of 50 + when women get closer to menopause, yoni mudrā gives much-needed relief from pain and cramps.

For pregnancy this mudrā is done for 10 minutes every day. This helps in a painless natural delivery. (Prāṇa mudrā and yoni mudrā)

Svasa (Asthma) Mudrā

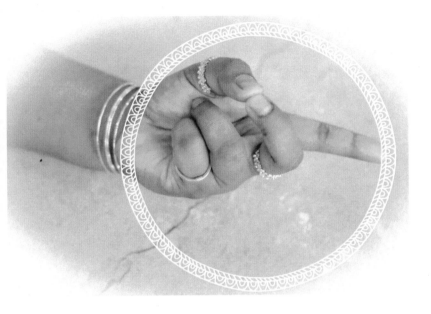

Place the tips of the little finger and ring to the base of the thumb. Now touch the tip of your middle finger to the tip of the thumb. Let the index finger be free and thrust forward.

Benefits :

For those with asthma, practice this mudrā in both hands for 15-20 minutes, it gives tremendous relief.

Vajra Mudrā

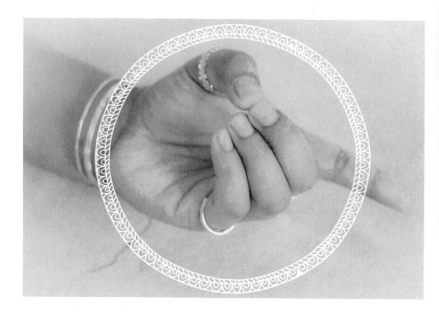

Press the tip of the thumb to the tip of the middle finger. Keep the forefinger open. Hold the ring and little finger as shown.

Benefits : When the earth principle becomes weak in the body, a person suffers from low blood pressure and improper flow in the stomach, spleen, heart, and pancreas. Lack of interest, tiredness and concussions are common on such occasions.

When practiced regularly, Vajra mudrā detoxes the excretory organs and lightens the body. Officegoers will find it very beneficial.

Mahaseersha Mudrā

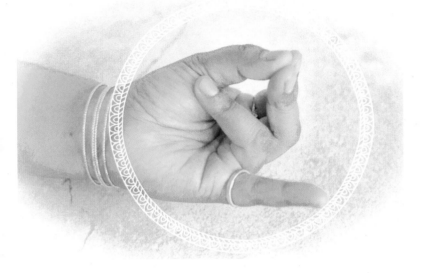

Touch the index and middle fingers to the tip of the thumb. Place the ring finger in the middle of the hand and press the base of the thumb softly. Stretch the small finger.

Change in the environment or stress may weaken our digestion leading to accumulation of waste in the body and mind. This may bring about stress and pain in the head, eyes, and the back. The main cause is lack of proper digestion.

This mudrā removes pain from the parts of the body by detoxing the body of the accumulated waste.

Shakti Mudrā

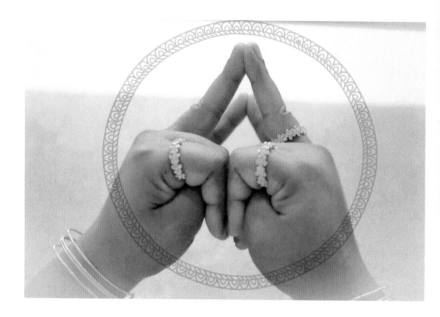

Touch the tips of ring finger and small finger of both hands. Thumbs are thrust to the middle of the hand. Now, hold the thumbs tightly with the index and middle fingers.

Benefits

Regulates respiratory activity above the stomach. It loosens hardness in the intestines and regulates the menstrual cycles among women giving them peace and sound sleep.

Sequence for detox mudrās

1. Sit in a comfortable position.
2. Join the hands in Namaste mudra at the top of your head.
3. Praying to the universal energy connect to the life of the universe. Keep back straight.
4. Bring the hands in front of your chest and hold them in a prayer position. Now follow with sequence given below.
5. Śaṅkha Mudrā
6. Sahaj Śaṅkha Mudrā
7. Hakini mudrā (Feel the pulse in all fingers)- 3 minutes
8. Makara mudrā (Heal the kidneys) - 4 minutes
9. Matangi mudrā (Heal the excretory system)- 4 minutes
10. Vajra mudrā (Heal the digestive system) - 4 minutes
11. Svasa mudrā (Heal the lungs) - 4 minutes
12. *Prāṇa* mudrā (energize the body) - 5 minutes
13. Meditate on your body healing through the practice.
14. Join your palms and end with a prayer.

Sequence for Menstrual cycle healing

1. Sit in a comfortable position.
2. Bring the hands in front of your chest and hold them in a prayer position. Now follow with sequence given below.
3. Matangi mudrā (Heal the excretory system)- 4 minutes
4. Shakti mudrā (Heal the pelvic region) - 8 minutes
5. Yoni mudrā (Heal the pelvic region) - 8 minutes
6. *Prāṇa* mudrā (energize the body) - 5 minutes
7. Join your palms and end with a prayer

Mudrā for Life

Life is full of desires. These desires can be fulfilled when we are focussed, calm and work in the right direction. We need physical and mental efficiency. In mudrās for life we begin with a sequence for calming down. This sequence is meant to heal you after a long tired day at work, or when you need to simply calm down.

We also have the next sequence to help you visualize your dream. Break it down to achievable goals and then enthusiastically achieve them. We need enthusiasm and proper planning. This visualization meditation is meant to help you achieve this goal.

Finally we have a series of mudrās for deeper meditation.

 please checkout the audio and video of the sequences on our website: www.yoginataraj.com/mudra

Meditation Sequence - 1

For Calming down

Sit down in a comfortable position. You can sit in any proper easy sitting position keeping back erect.

1. Awareness on your breathing. Begin with the focus on your throat. As you breathe in and out cast away all other points of focus and meditate exclusively on the sound of your breath.
2. As you focus on your breath observe your breath advance deeper and deeper. The sound of your own breath is healing to the body. It is called oceanic breath because it sounds like a beautiful soothing ocean wave.
3. Meditation begins with purification of the energy channels and the mind by performing the Śaṅkha mudrā. Perform Śaṅkha mudrā keeping hands in front of your chest. Breathe deeply and only focus on your breath for the next 3 minutes.
4. Now perform Sahaj Śaṅkha mudrā for 5 minutes.
4. Now Ganesha mudrā to take a vow. Meditate on Lord Ganesha, perform the Ganesha mudrā. Take a vow that "I will calm down, I vow to throw away all anger, I vow to forgive and forget, I will heal. O Ganesha, kindly remove all obstacles that hinder my path to peace."
5. After taking the vow now perform the Gyān mudrā. As you practice the Gyān mudrā focus on the breath only. Meditate on the beautiful rising sun. Feel as though your breath is like a wave of an ocean producing a beautiful sound.

Step 6. Meditate on the rising sun, the beautiful sound of the breath and practice the gyāna mudrā for 20 minutes. Simply bathe in the refreshing sound of your breath. Feel refreshed and relaxed.

Step 7: Now perform Hākini Mudrā. Remember all the beautiful things experienced for 5 minutes.

Step 8. Focus on your heart, be grateful, chant Om 3 times and relax.

Meditation Sequence - 2

Sit down in a comfortable position. You can sit in any proper easy sitting position keeping back erect.

1. Focus on your breathing. Begin with the focus on your throat. As you breathe in and out cast away all other points of focus and meditate exclusively on the sound of your breath.

2. As you focus on your breath observe your breath advance deeper and deeper. Imagine as if your applying the healing oinmtment of your own breath to the self. It is called oceanic breath because it sounds like a beautiful soothing ocean wave.

3. Meditation begins with purification of the energy channels and the mind by performing the Śaṅkha mudrā. Perform Śaṅkha mudrā keeping hands in front of your chest. Clasp the left thumb with the fingers of the right hand. Breathe

deeply and only focus on your breath for the next 3 minutes.

4. After Śaṅkha mudrā perform the Ganesha mudrā to take a vow. Meditate on Lord Ganesha, perform the Ganesha mudrā. Take a vow that "I will calm down, I vow to focus on the task to acheive success in my task. O Ganesha, kindly remove all obstacles that hinder our path to success."

5. After taking the vow perform the Gyāna mudrā. Focus on your mind, purge all the thoughts and let only one thought remain, i.e your purpose, nothing else.

6. Focus on the beginning , middle and end of the goal.

7. Meditate on the steps needed to achieve your goal.

8. Focus on the timeline.

9. Meditate on how you achieve it in the present situation.

10. Make room for the progress, meditate on the best possible solution.

11. Meditate on the universal energy, and pray for the energy to be with you and guide you in your goal.

12. Now revisit your goal and your steps. Strengthen your mind.

13. Visualize practically how your goal is achieved.

14. Focus on your heart, be grateful and chant Om 3 times and relax.

15. This practice will make you feel positive/enthusiastic and enlivened.

Meditation Sequence - 3

For Deep Meditation

Sit down in a comfortable position. You can sit in any proper easy sitting position keeping back erect.

1. Let's focus on breathing. Begin with focus on your throat. As you breathe in and out cast away all other points of focus and meditate exclusively on the sound of your breath.
2. As you focus on your breath observe your breath go deeper and deeper.
3. As you focus on your breath observe your breath advance deeper and deeper. The sound of your own breath is healing to the body. It is called oceanic breath because it sounds like a beautiful soothing ocean wave.
4. Meditation begins with purification of the energy channels and the mind by performing the Śaṅkha mudrā.
5. Now perform Sahaj Śaṅkha mudrā
6. After Śaṅkha mudrā practice the Ganesha mudrā to take a vow. Meditate on Lord Ganesha, perform the Ganesha mudrā. Take a vow that "I will calm down, I vow to release away all anger, I vow to forgive and forget, I will heal. O Ganesha, kindly remove all obstacles that hinder my path to peace."
7. Perform the Karana Mudrā. Meditate on your inner strength. Focus on removing all those forces that are hindering your progress. Meditate that all negative forces and

obstacles are all gone.

8. Perform the Dharmachakra mudrā. Meditate on the beautiful workings of nature. The rising of sun, the rising of the moon. The beautiful seasons, all the beautiful fruits and trees. Meditate on the beautiful flowing rivers and the variety of species in all respects. Meditate on the beautiful sky and realize the depth and beauty of the sky.

9. Perform Ksepana mudrā and focus on the hands meditating on the nectar of immortality. Meditate on the region of the heart and feel the increase of healing nectar and the nectar of immortality.

10. Perform Samana mudrā to balance all the elements.

11. Meditate on yourself filled up with energy and the mind fully calm and healthy ready for a higher realization.

12. Focus on your heart, be grateful and chant Om 3 times and relax

To video and practice along with Yogi Nataraj please visit

www.yoginataraj.com/mudra

Mudrās for Therapy

Here is a list of the most common ailments alphabetically and we have given a list of mudrās that can be practiced.

To video videos of these mudras please visit
www.yoginataraj.com/mudra

Anxiety

20 Minutes Vāyu Mudrā (27)
20 Minutes Gyāna Mudrā (29)

Arthiritis

10 Minutes Vāyu Mudrā (27)
10 minutes Vāta Nāshak (49)
10 minutes Prithvi Vardhak
10 Minutes Apāna Vāyu Mudrā (62)

Alzheimer's

20 minutes Gyān Mudrā (29)
20 minutes Vāta Kārak Mudrā (50)

Acidity

15 minutes Prithvi-Mudrā (41)
15 minutes Prāṇa Mudrā (52)
15 minutes Jāl-shāmak (44)

Anemia

20 minutes Varun Mudrā (46)
10 minutes Āakāsh-Mudrā (35)

Anger

10 minuutes Gyāna-Mudrā (29)
10 minutes Prithvi-Mudrā (37)
10 minutes Prāṇa Mudrā (52)

Asthma

15 min Linga mudrā (68)
15 min Āakāsh-Mudrā (35)
15 min Svasa Mudrā (89)

Allergy

15 min Śaṅkha mudrā (71)
15 min Prithvi-vardhak (41)

Also Follow the Detox mudrā series

Bradycardia

40 minutes Gyān Mudrā (29)

Breathlessness

40 minutes Vāyu Mudrā (27)

Bone Strengthening

40 minutes Prithvi-Mudrā (41)

Backache

20 minutes Vāyu Mudrā (27)
10 minutes Apāna- vāyu (
10 minutes Vāta-nāshak

Blood Pressure (If high)

10 minutes Ākāsh-Mudrā
10 minutes Prāṇa mudrā (52)
10 minutes Apāna- vāyu (60)
10 minutes Vāta-kārak (50)

Blood Pressure (if low)

20 minutes Prithvi-vardhak (41)
20 minutes Sūnya Mudrā (33)

C Constipation

10 minutes Vāyu Mudrā (27)
10 minutes Vāta-nāshak mudrā (49)
10 minutes Prithvi- shāmak or Sūrya mudrā (38)
10 minutes Jal –vardhak or Varun mudrā (46)

Chronic fatigue

20 minutes Prithvi mudrā (41)
20 minutes Vāta-nāshak mudrā (49)
10 minutes Prāṇa mudrā (52)

Cervical spondylosis

20 minutes Vāta-nāshak mudrā (49)
10 minutes Varun mudrā (46)
10 minutes Prithvi mudrā (41)
10 minutes Apān- vāyu mudrā (62)

Cramps (muscles)

20 minutes Varun mudrā (46)
20 minutes Vāyu Mudrā (27)

Depression

20 minutes Gyāna mudrā (29)
10 minutes Prithvi mudrā (41)
10 minutes Prāṇa mudrā (52)

Dementia

20 minutes Gyāna mudrā (29)
20 minutes Hākini mudrā (83)

Diabetes Mellitus

20 minutes Gyāna mudrā (29)
10 minutes Apāna mudrā (60)
10 minutes Prāṇa mudrā (52)

Deaf (Hearing loss)

10 minutes Ākāsh-Mudrā (35)
10 minutes Sūnya Mudrā (33)

Dehydration & Hormonal Imbalance

40 minutes Jal —vardhak or Varun mudrā (46)

Diarrhea

10 min Jal-shāmak mudrā (44)
10 min Apān mudrā (60)
10 min Vāta-kārak or Vāyān mudrā (50)
10 min Prithvi mudrā (41)

E Eye Ailments

If eyes are too watery

15 minutes Sūrya mudrā (38)
15 minutes Kapha-nāshak mudrā (51)

For Glaucoma

40 minutes Jal-shāmak mudrā (44)

F Fear

15 minutes Gyāna mudrā (29)
15 minutes Ākāsh mudrā (35)
10 minutes Vāta-nāshak mudrā

Flatulance

15 minutes Vāyu mudrā (27)
15 minutes Vāta-nāshak mudrā (49)
10 minutes Apān mudrā (60)

Frozen shoulder

20 minutes Vāyu mudrā (27)
20 minutes Apān mudrā (60)

Fracture Healing

40 minutes Prithvi mudrā (41)

G Gastritis

15 minutes Prithvi mudrā (41)
15 minutes Apān mudrā (60)
15 minutes Varuna mudrā (46)

Greying of hair/Gastric ulcer

20 minutes Prithvi mudrā (41)
20 minutes Prāṇa mudrā (52)
10 minutes Varuna mudrā

Hyperacidity

20 minutes Prithvi mudrā (41)
10 minutes Jal Shāmak mudrā (44)
10 minutes Prāṇa mudrā (52)

Headache

10 minutes Apān- vāyu mudrā (62)
10 minutes Vāta-nāshak mudrā (49)
10 minutes Vāyu mudrā (27)

I Inflammation

20 minutes Prāṇa mudrā (52)
20 minutes Prithivi mudrā (41)

Indigestion

10 minutes Sūrya mudrā (38)
10 minutes Linga mudrā (68)
10 minutes Kapha Nāshak mudrā (51)
10 minutes Varun mudrā

Infertility

20 minutes Prithivi mudrā (41)
20 minutes Kapha Kārak mudrā (52)
10 minutes Varun mudrā (46)

Insomnia

20 minutes Vāyu mudrā (27)
10 minutes Prāṇa mudrā (52)
10 minutes Prithivi mudrā (41)

J Joint Pains

20 minutes Vāyu mudrā (27)
20 minutes Prithivi mudrā (41)
10 minutes Apān- vāyu mudrā (62)

K Kidney Ailments

10 minutes Apān- vāyu mudrā (62)
10 minutes Apāna mudrā (60)
10 minutes Jal Shāmak mudrā (44)

L Liver Ailments

20 minutes Sūrya mudrā (38)
20 minutes Linga mudrā (68)

M Muscle strengthening

20 minutes Shankha mudrā (71)
20 minutes Gyāna mudrā (29)

Muscle Spasms

20 minutes Vāyu mudrā (27)
20 minutes Varun mudrā (46)

Memory

20 minutes Gyāna mudrā (29)
20 minutes Prithivi mudrā (41)
10 minutes Prāṇa mudrā (52)

Migraine

20 minutes Gyāna mudrā (29)
10 minutes Apān mudrā (60)
15 minutes Ākāsh mudrā (35)

Menstrual

Excess
20 minutes Prithivi mudrā (41)
10 minutes Yoni mudrā 87)
10 minutes Shankha mudrā (71)
10 minutes Jal Shāmak mudrā (44)
Too little
20 minutes Sūrya mudrā (38)
10 minutes Varun mudrā (46)
10 minutes Shakti mudrā (92)
10 minutes *Prāṇa* mudrā (52)

N Nose

Loss of smell
40 minutes Prithivi mudrā (41)

Runny Nose
40 minutes Jal Shāmak mudrā (44)

Nose Blocked
20 minutes Sūrya mudrā (38)
20 minutes Kapha nāsak mudrā (51)

Nausea

20 minutes Vāyu mudrā (27)
10 minutes Apān mudrā (60)

Obesity

20 minutes Sūrya mudrā (38)
20 Minutes Vāyān mudrā (50)

Parkinson's

20 minutes Vāyu mudrā (27)
20 minutes Apān Vāyu mudrā (62)
10 minutes Gyāna mudrā (29)

Psoriasis

20 minutes Vāyu mudrā (27)
20 minutes Varun mudrā (46)

Piles

20 minutes Prithivi mudrā (41)
10 minutes Apān Vāyu mudrā (62)
10 minutes Apān mudrā (60)

S Stress/Sciatica

20 minutes Vāyu mudrā (27)
20 minutes Vāta nāsak mudrā(49)

Skin dry

20 minutes Prana mudrā (52)
10 minutes Prithivi mudrā (41)
10 minutes Varuna mudrā (46)

Sweating

If Excessive Sweating/Swelling
20 minutes Prithivi mudrā (41)
20 minutes Jal Shāmak mudrā (44)

If no sweat
20 minutes Sūrya mudrā (38)
20 minutes *Prāṇa* mudrā (52)

Stammering

10 minutes Vāta nāsak mudrā (49)
15 minutes Śaṅkha mudrā (71)
15 minutes Sahaj Śaṅkha mudrā (73)

Taste Issues
40 minutes Varun mudrā (46)

Thyroid

Underactive
10 minutes Sūrya mudrā (38)
10 minutes Kapha nāsak mudrā (51)
10 minutes Linga mudrā (68)
10 minutes Prāṇa mudrā (52)

Overactive
20 minutes Prithvi mudrā (41)
20 minutes Vāyu mudrā (27)
10 minutes Prāṇa mudrā (52)

Tooth Ache

20 minutes Vāta nāsak mudrā (49)
20 minutes Apān Vāyu mudrā (62)

Ulcers

20 minutes Prithvi mudrā (41)
20 minutes Prāṇa mudrā (52)

Voice Improvement

40 minutes Gyāna mudrā (29)
15 minutes Śaṅkha mudrā (71)
15 minutes Sahaj Śaṅkha mudrā (73)

Vertigo

20 minutes Vāyu mudrā (27)
20 minutes Vāta nāsak mudrā (49)

Vericose veins

20 minutes Prithvi mudrā (41)
20 minutes Apān Vāyu mudrā (62)

W Weight Loss

Follow the weight loss series (39)

W Weight Gain

20 minutes Prithvi mudrā (41)
10 minutes Apān mudrā (60)
10 minutes Prāṇa mudrā (52)

Water Retention

20 minutes Sūrya mudrā (38)
20 minutes Linga mudrā (68)
10 minutes Jal Shāmak mudrā (44)

Glossary of words

Nādis — subtle nerves

Vāta — Combination of air and Ether. Transport mechanism within the body

Pitta - Combination of water and fire. The chemical components in the body.

Kapha - Combination of water and earth. The physical components in the body.

Vāyu - Air

Gyāna — knowledge , to be in knowledge

Sunya — Zero

Ākasha -Ether , sky

Surya - Sun, Heat

Prithvi- Earth

Jal - Water

Shāmak — To reduce , control

Varuṇa — Water , ocean

Nāshaka - Destroy, Control

Pañcha- Five

Prāṇa - Energy Life air Prāṇa

Vyāna — Air which circulates around the body balancing the body.

Apāna - Downward air

Samāna — Air which supports Fire in the belly

Udana - Air in the neck region

Musti - closed fist

Ādi - First

Linga - Phallus symbol

Pushan — Heat Generating

Śaṅkha – Conch, a symbol of purity

Sahaj Śaṅkha – Easy conch mudra

Ganesha – Lord Ganesha who removes obstacles

Rudra – Lord Shiva

Dharma – Dharma means spiritual pinciples

Chakra – Wheel , circle

Karana - Cause

Dhyāna - Meditate

Kārak - Cause of

Mudrā Course with Yogi Nataraj

If you would like to learn this science of mudrās from Yogi Nataraj in person please visit www.yoginataraj.com/mudra and sign up for the course. We are offering a discount to all those who purchase this book. The discount code is yogisbook9 and you will get a 18% off on the course. This offer is for limited time only.

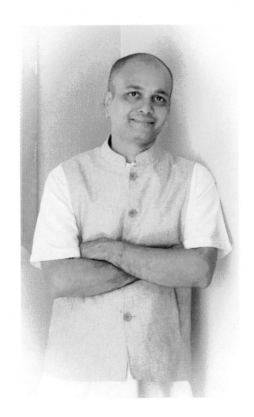

About the Author

Yogi Nataraj is an author, Astrologer, yoga consultant, Mudrā healer and specializes in philosophy and application of yoga. He is based in Las Vegas, USA and teaches this science across the world. He is also known for accurate readings in astrology. Along with his wife Sundari Dasi, he conducts courses in Ayurveda, Mudra healing, meditation and Yoga teacher training.

His contact information is as follows

Whatsapp : +17029563123

Facebook : https://www.facebook.com/yoginataraj9

Website : www.yoginataraj.com

Email : info@yoginataraj.com

DISCLAIMER

Mudrā therapy is not a substitute for prescribed treatment or medications for illnesses. The book is for your information and you are must consult your doctor and a professional mudrā healer before making any changes to treatment. The author and the book accept no liability for injury or damage resulting from your decision to use the information or instruction in this book or our website.

We have given you the best information after lot of research. Please use this information responsibly after due consideration and consultation with professionals.

Our aim is to spread this Yogic knowledge to all, for everyones benefit. Thank you.

Made in United States
Orlando, FL
04 January 2024

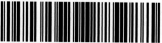

42147852R00069